EVAN YVONNE

IT'S A GIRL THING...

TEEN RETREAT BOOK

facilitators guide

Dear Facilitators,

Thank you for your willingness to be a facilitator of the It's A Girl Thing Movement! Your love and desire to serve young women believers is precious and we appreciate the work you do.

We are living in a culture where girls are evolving and we have a great opportunity to help them identify and navigate through all the choices in life with grace, dignity, poise- but mostly, in the fear and admonition of our Lord. Our girls must be different. They must be those who are willing to uphold the standards of God- unapologetically while gaining the favor of both God and men.

This retreat book is full of opportunities for you as the facilitator to open up questions and dialogue for the girls. You have the liberty to freestyle and add in games, journaling, or other activities to bring their experience out into safe spaces.

We invite you to give feedback or send us clips of your event with testimonials! Please follow us on our YouTube channel @ministryalliancelove

QUICK TIPS:

- Create digital parent/guardian permission slips
- host event at a hotel/resort that has an on-site restaurant and spa
- Request a pre-order menu (limited menu) for all dining experiences
- Use a commercial name for in-room buffet catering or supply items that are basic, like Pizza and veggie tray.
- encourage girls to journal their experience as often as possible and/or as soon as they finish an activity
- Create a video journal log space to give an option of journaling that they are willing to share.
- Ask facilitators to video journal their experience as well
- Create a short video presentation with pictures and testimonies for girls (parents) to have as a keepsake.

SUGGESTED ITINERARY SCHEDULE

DAY CONFERENCE VERSION

- **hold the conference at an entertainment complex, theme park, modern bowling alley, or space where food and activities are available**

SESSION ONE

9am: Icebreaker Game

9:15: Body Changes discussion and journaling

9:30: Snacks and Boys, Boys, Boys

11am: Break for an activity at the venue

12 noon: lunch

SESSION TWO

1pm: Beauty and Hygiene

2pm: Self-Care

3pm: Break for an activity at the venue and snacks

4:30pm: Family

5:30 pm: Pick-up

SUGGESTED ITINERARY SCHEDULE
SLEEP OVER VERSION

DAY ONE:
4-5pm: Meet and greet hot chocolate bar mixer
5:15-6:15pm: Body Changes
6:30-7:45pm: Dinner Buffet (in-room)
8:00- 9pm: Boys, Boys, Boys
9:30-12 midnight: Movie

DAY TWO:
7:30-9:30am: Breakfast and Dining Etiquette
9:45-11:30am: Beauty and Hygiene
12 noon-1:30pm: Lunch
1:45-3pm: Self Care/Armor of God
3:15-5:30pm: Spa Activity
5:45-6:45pm: Family part 1
7:30-9:30pm: Fancy Dinner
10:00-12 midnight: Movie

DAY THREE:
7:30-8:30am: Breakfast and the Word
8:45-10:30am: Family Part 2
10:40- 11am: Pick-Up

TABLE OF CONTENTS

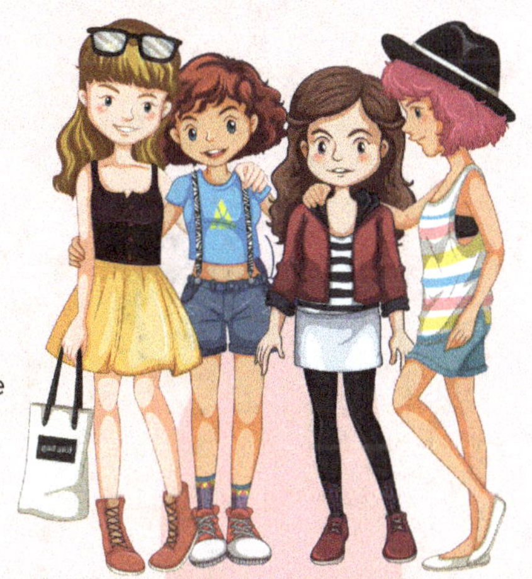

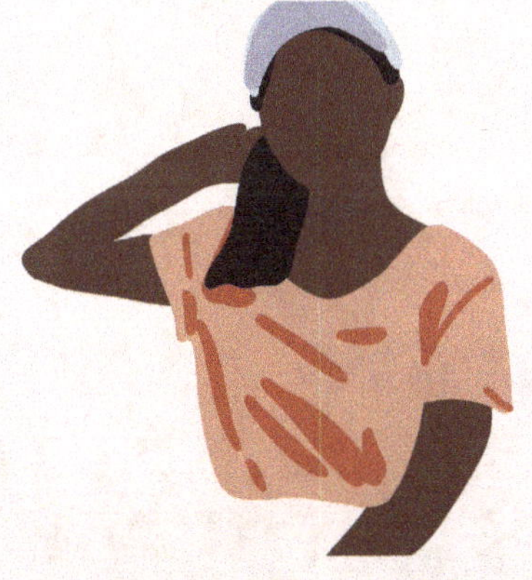

Psalms 32:8- "I will guide you along the best pathway for your life."

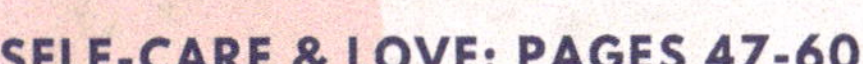

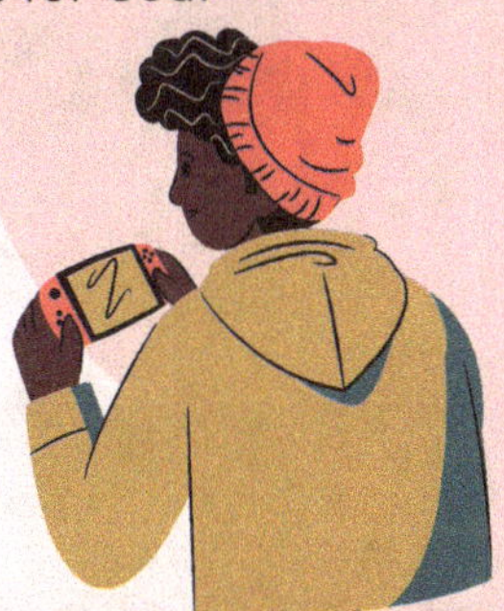

Section 1

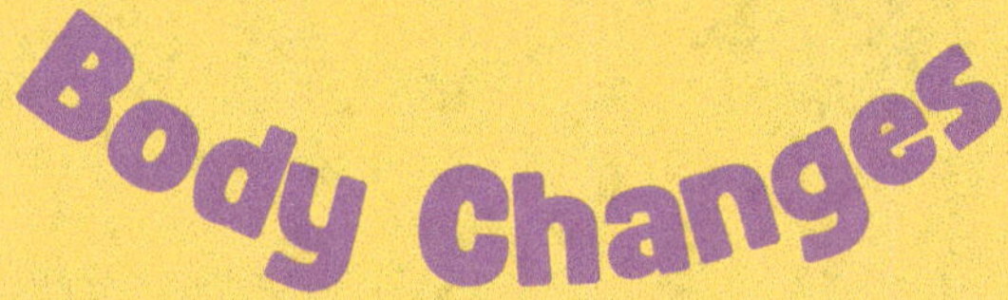

UP HERE & DOWN THERE

UP HERE...

Face: as girls grow older, our facial features become more enhanced and there are so many ways too embrace the changes;

- Follow influencers who look like you. Seeing a positive image of someone who looks like you can help you become more comfortable with trying new looks or just being comfortable in your skin.

- Make time to embrace your natural self. Looking in the mirror doesn't have to be vain- it's a great way to accept the way you look and build confidence in what you actually like about yourself.

Hair: as you grow older, it's totally natural to want to try different types of hair styles to express your character. Some hair choices may actually make you look older so it's best to stay away from super mature hairstyles. Fun rinse out hair colors or extensions are great ways to add a little flair to your maturing image. Make sure your parents are comfortable with what you would like to do- parent support is the key to exploring new looks as you grow older.

Breasts: Breasts are great but they have a purpose; to produce milk to feed your children when you have them. As they grow, you get more attention from both girls and boys. Make sure that if anyone is making you feel uncomfortable about your body growths that you speak up. Tell them that

what they are saying is uncomfortable and you don't like it. If the comments don't stop, get an adult to help you communicate with the offender.
Once you begin to realize that your breasts are growing, grab your mom or an aunt and ask them to take you shopping for bra's! Make a fun date out of it by going to get lunch or lattes once the shopping is complete!
The best way to embrace growing breasts is to get excited that God has equipped you with the feeding solution to help your baby grow healthy during the first years of her life! Until that day comes- your job is to simply take care of your breasts.

DISCUSSION: WHAT CHANGES ARE YOUR FACE AND SKIN GOING THROUGH AS YOU GET OLDER? WHAT ARE SOME WAYS THAT YOU EMBRACE THOSE CHANGES? WHAT DO YOU LIKE ABOUT THE IMAGE THAT YOU PROJECT?

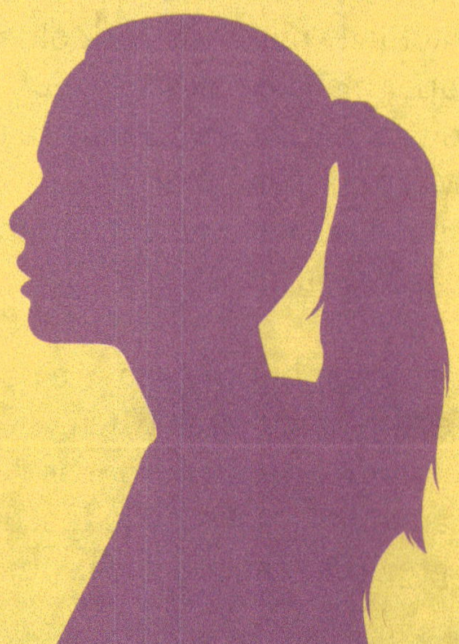

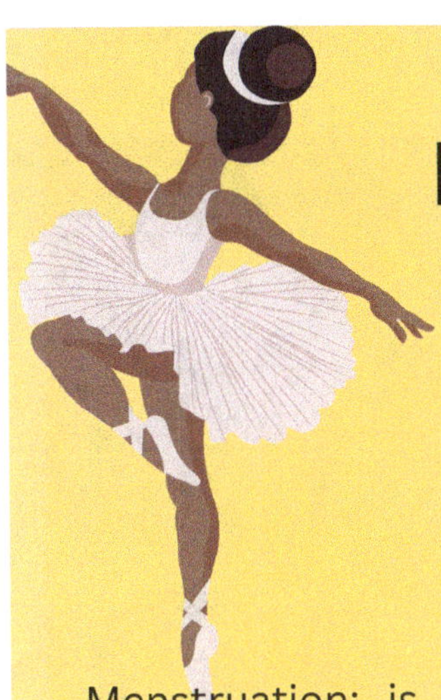

DOWN THERE...

Now all of us have become like one who is unclean. And all of our righteous deeds are like a filthy garment. And all of us wither like a leaf. And all of our iniquities take us away.

ISAIAH 64:6

Menstruation: is a monthly cycle that rids the body of impurities through the flowing of blood. Once your menstrual cylcle begins, you are able to conceive a child. Metaphorically, menstruation represents sin (as we read in the passage above. The Good News is that Jesus satisfied all laws and rituals associated with a woman's monthly cycle. We are no longer unclean and impure in God's eyes- we are redeemed and a new creation in Christ!

Biologically, we understand that having a monthly cycle lets your body know that you can start making a family; conceiving a child, carrying a child in your womb, and delivering a child. This monthly cycle may come with discomfort and bad mood vibes. The best way to help yourself during your cycle is to drink lots of water, remain active, and practice patience and kindness with yourself and toward others.

Your potential to become a mother is something to celebrate and look forward to when the time is right.

DISCUSSION:
- How can you honor God once you start menstruating?

- Are you looking forward to becoming a mother? What kind of mother would you like to be?

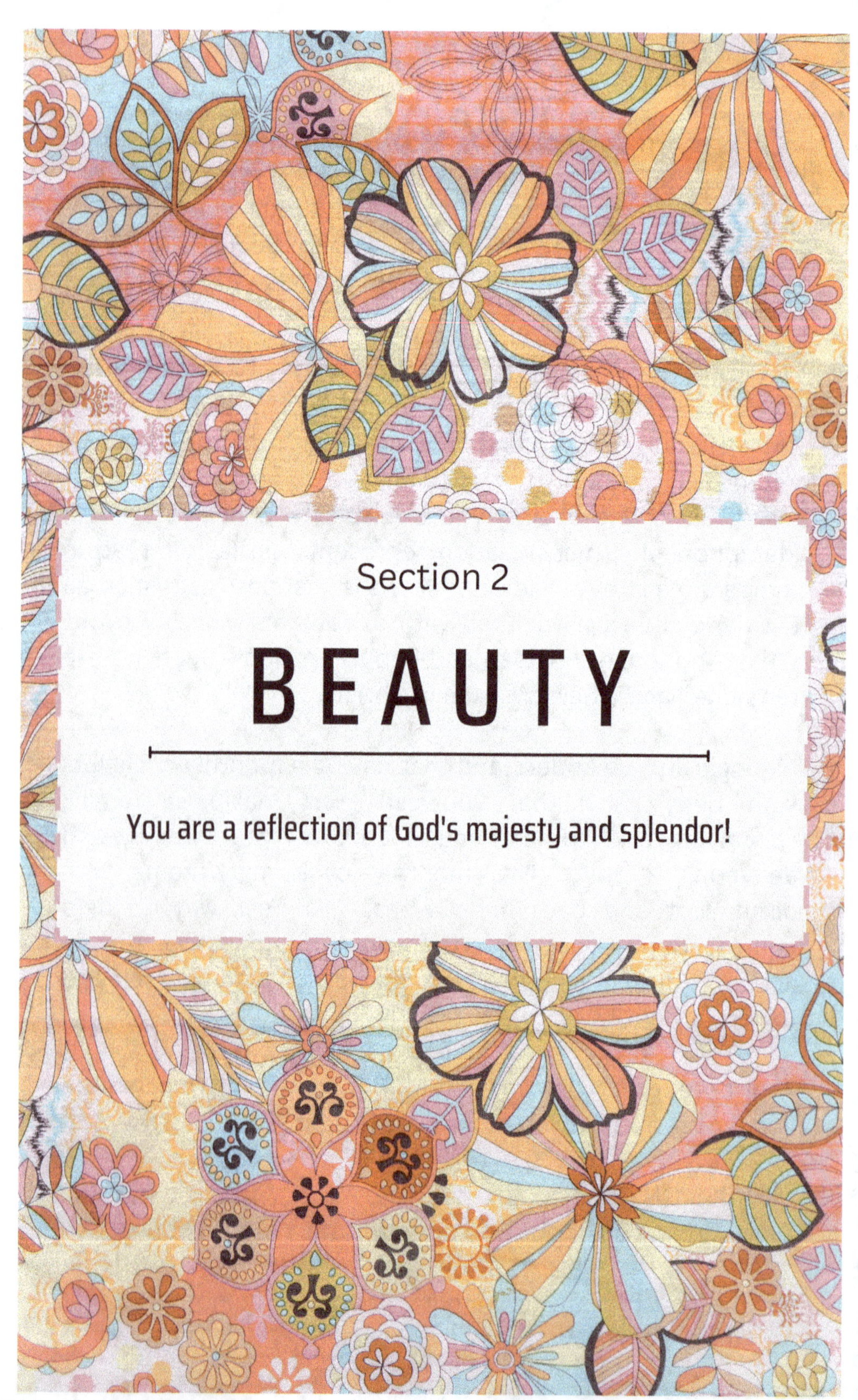

Section 2

BEAUTY

You are a reflection of God's majesty and splendor!

On the day you were born your umbilical cord was not cut, you weren't bathed and cleaned up, you weren't rubbed with salt, you weren't wrapped in a baby blanket. No one cared a fig for you. No one did one thing to care for you tenderly in these days. You were thrown out into a vacant lot and left there, dirty and unwashed- a newborn nobody wanted.
And then I came by. I saw you all miserable and bloody. Yes, I said to you, lying there helpless and filthy, Live! Grow up like a plant in the field!" And you did. You grew up. You grew tall and matured as a woman, full-breasted, with flowing hair. But you were naked and vulnerable, fragile and exposed.

I came by again and saw you, saw that you were ready for love and a lover. I took care of you, dressed you and protected you. I promised you my love and entered the covenant of marriage with you. I, God, the Master, gave my word. You became mine. I gave you a good bath, washing off all that old blood, and anointed you with aromatic oils. I dressed you in a colorful gown and put leather sandals on your feet. I gave you linen blouses and a fashionable wardrobe of expensive clothing.

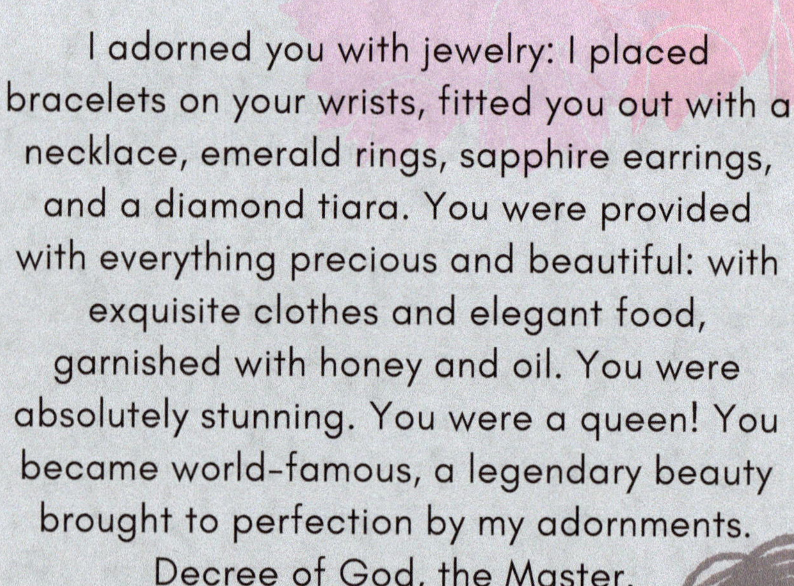

I adorned you with jewelry: I placed bracelets on your wrists, fitted you out with a necklace, emerald rings, sapphire earrings, and a diamond tiara. You were provided with everything precious and beautiful: with exquisite clothes and elegant food, garnished with honey and oil. You were absolutely stunning. You were a queen! You became world-famous, a legendary beauty brought to perfection by my adornments. Decree of God, the Master.

Ezekiel 16:4-16 MSG

stunning

YOU

are

who

God

says

YOU

are

brought to perfection

CROWNED WITH MAJESTY

a queen

Discussion:

1. What are some of the lies that you have believed about yourself?

2. If you are the baby in the story, what condition were you in when God found you?

3. What did God decide to do when he found you?

THE *Good*

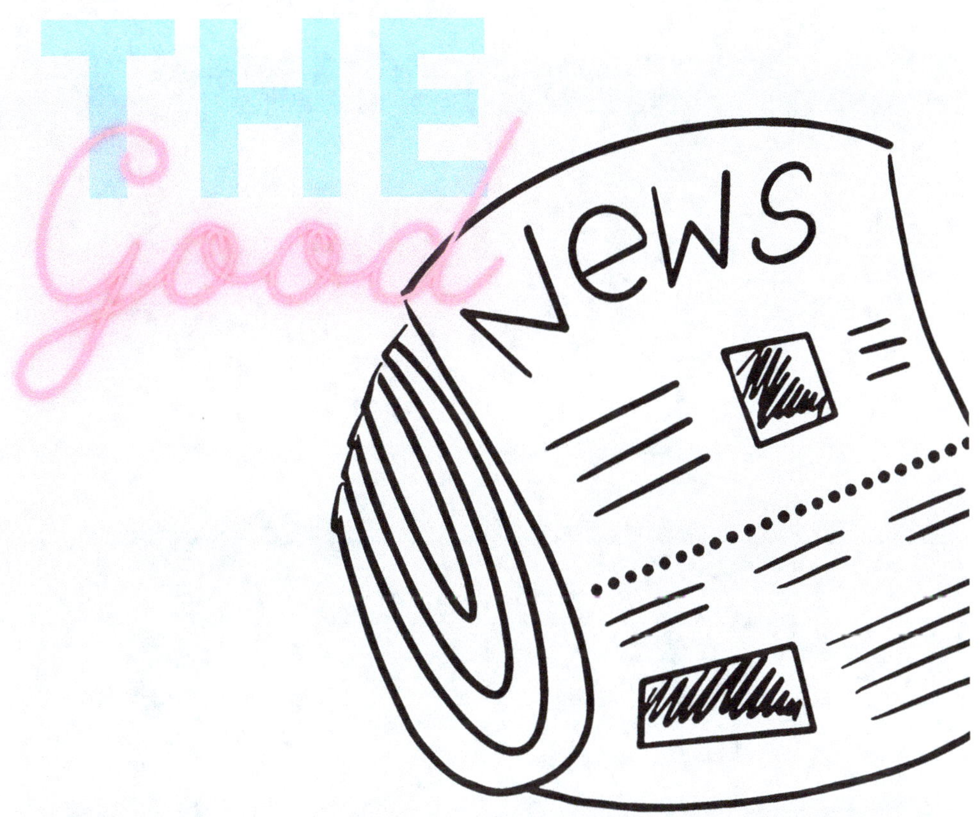

Ezekiel 16:63, I'll firmly establish my covenant with you and you'll know that I am God. You'll remember your past life and face the shame of it but when I make atonement for you, make everything right after all you have done, it will leave you speechless. Decree of God, the Master

Jesus is the atonement and fulfillment of God's new covenant with us. He firmly establishes our beauty and we should reflect the splendor and majesty of His kindness toward us!

...Our beauty is simply a
REFLECTION
MERCIFUL
LOVED
kind
PATIENT
fears God
HUMBLE

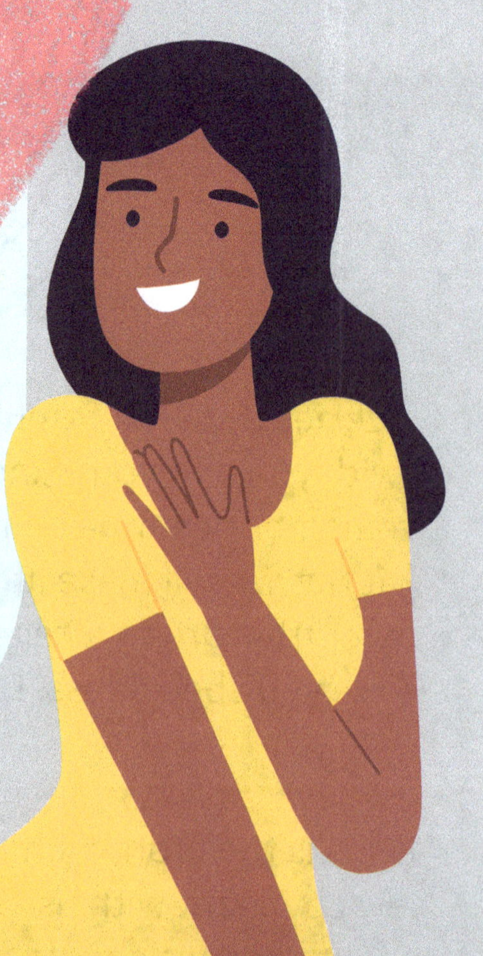

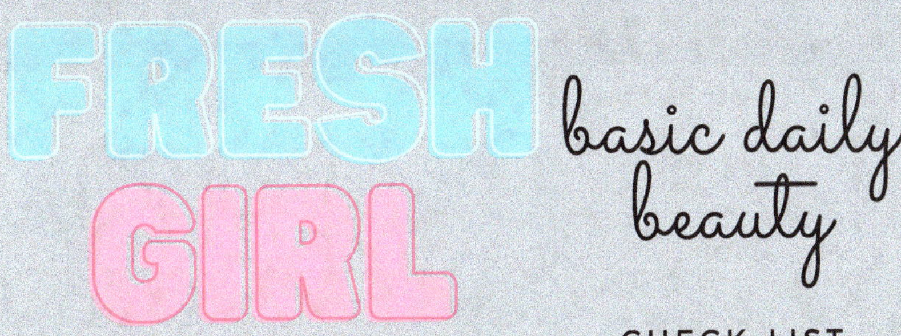

WASH: whether a bath or shower, make sure you have 2-washclothes for body and face, a natural soap, and a scrubber if you like to finish with smooth skin.

AFTER-WASH: a natural lotion, deodorant, toothpaste and tooth brush, body spray, and lip balm

FOR SCHOOL: pack a small cosmetic bag with a mini-brush, gel, edge cream, mini deodorant, floss, hair bands, sanitary napkins, feminine wipes, and a mini lotion to get you through the day. Keep this bag stashed in your locker!

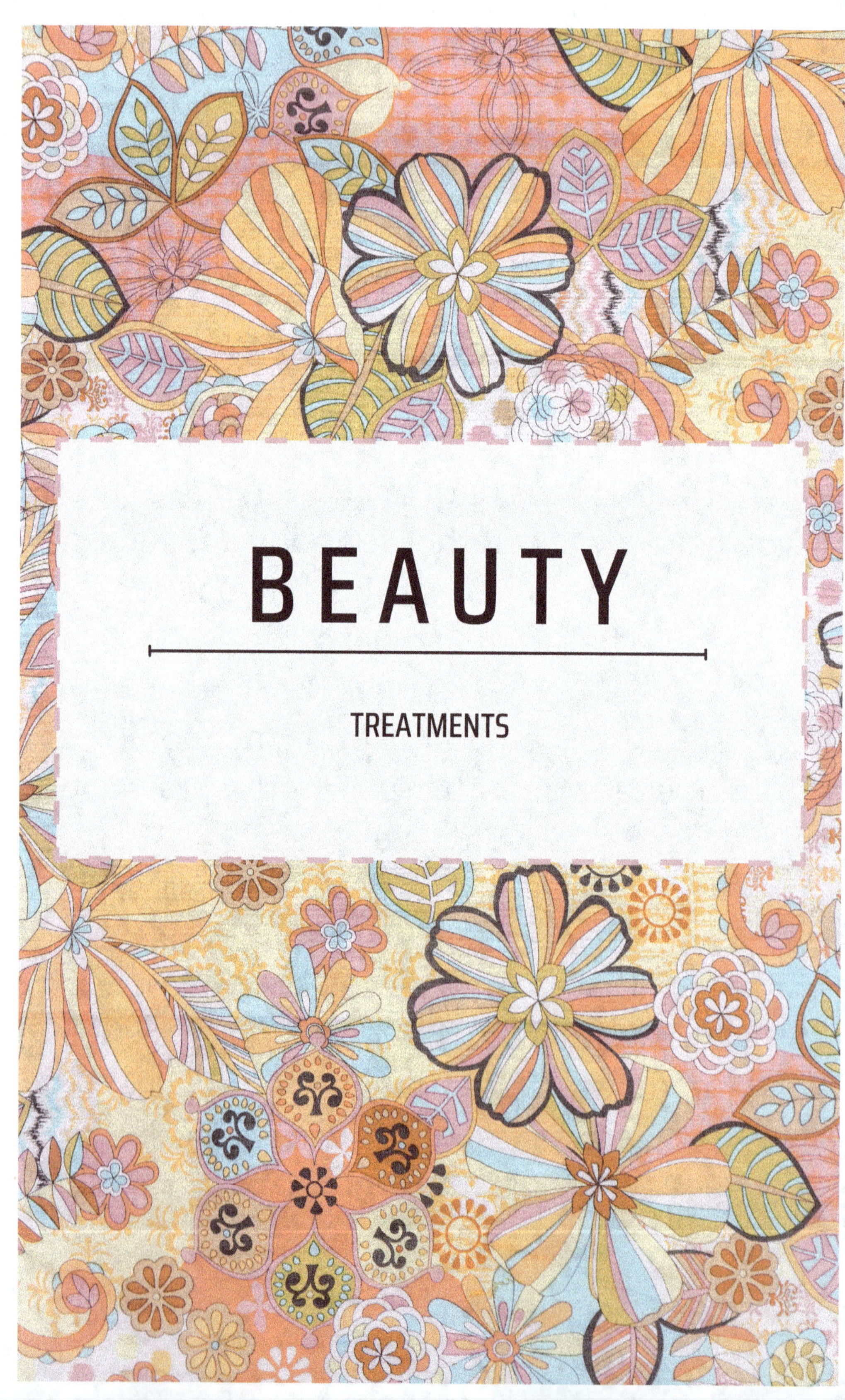
BEAUTY
TREATMENTS

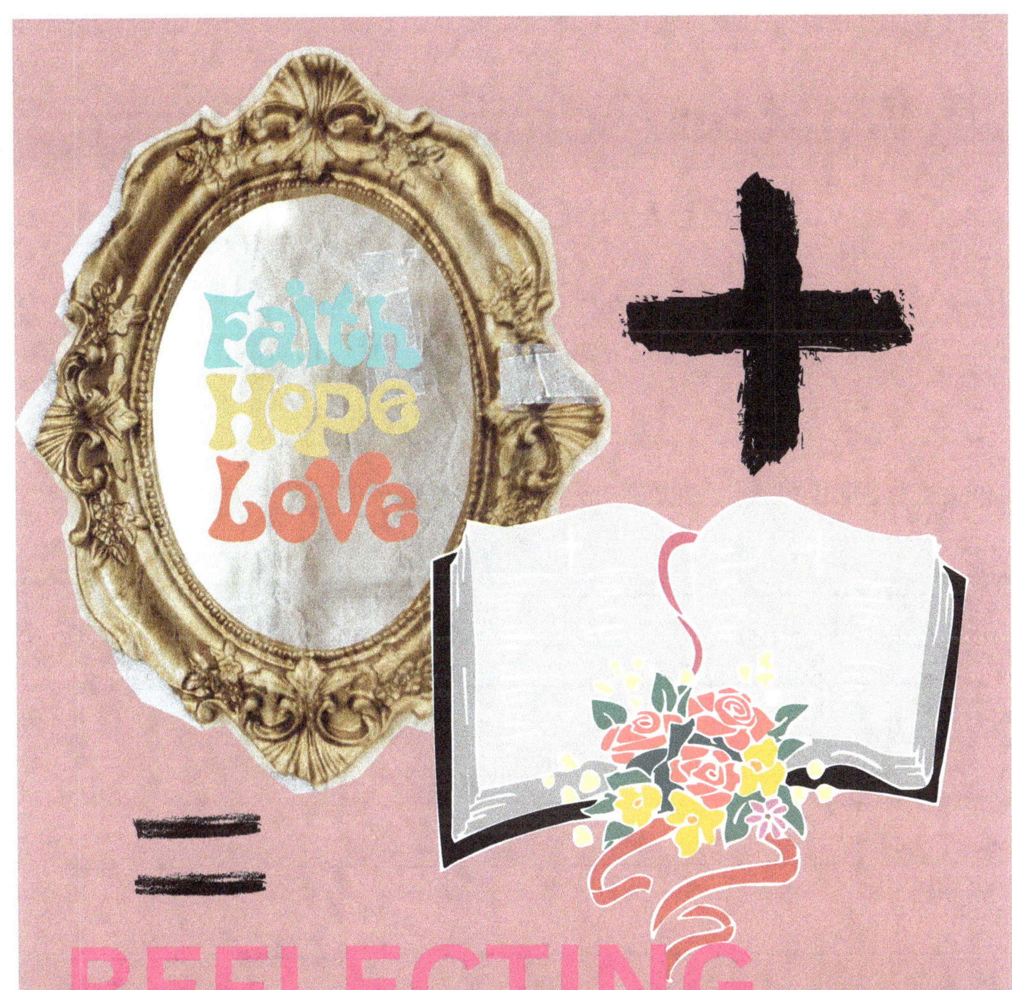

Faith
Hope
Love
REFLECTING
God's beauty means
that we must be
reading
HIS WORD
everyday!

What are some unique ways that God made you?

Think about the things that he placed inside of you that make you- you. Are you artistic, sporty, inquisitive, laid-back?

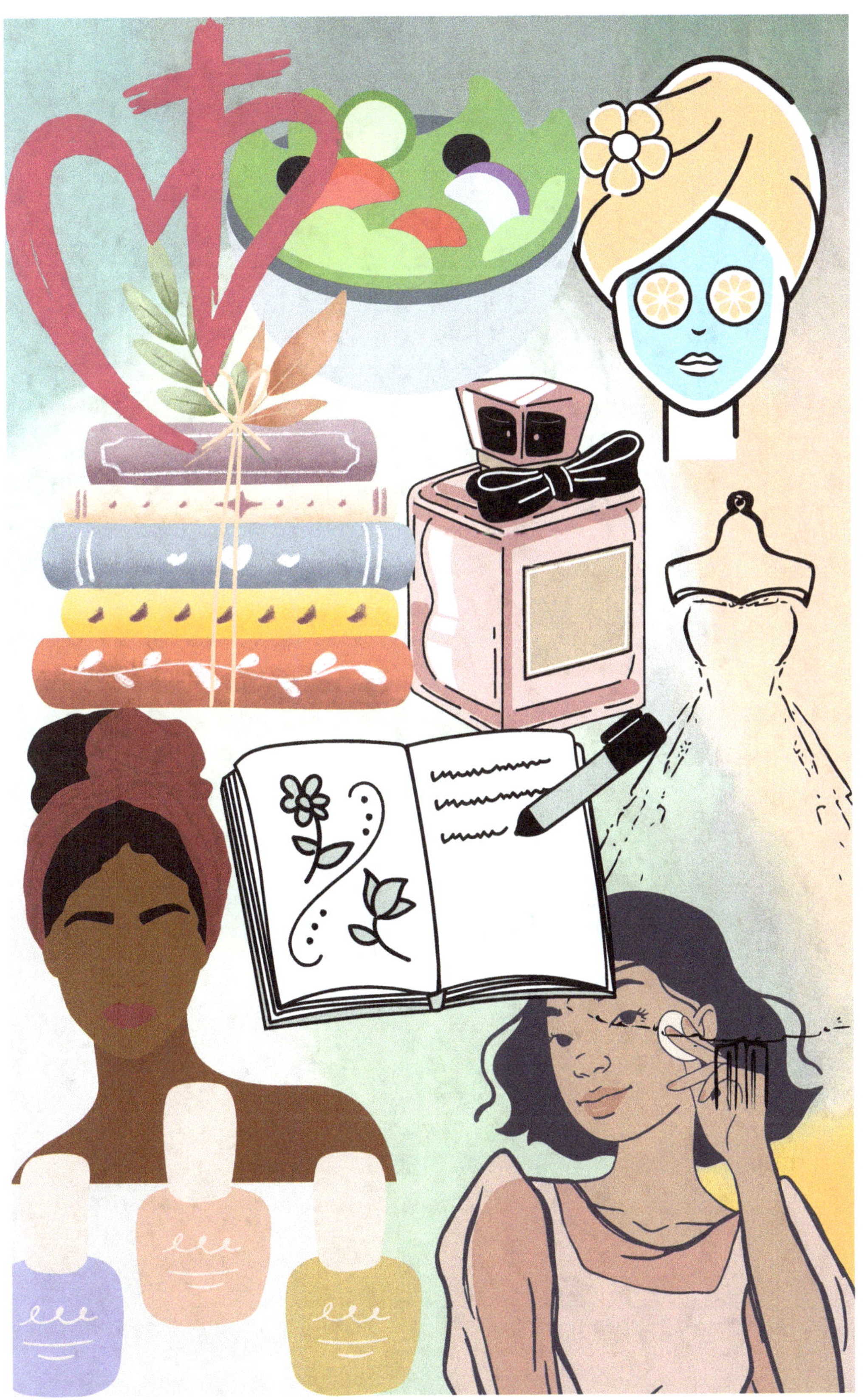

In what ways can you take care of who God created you to be?

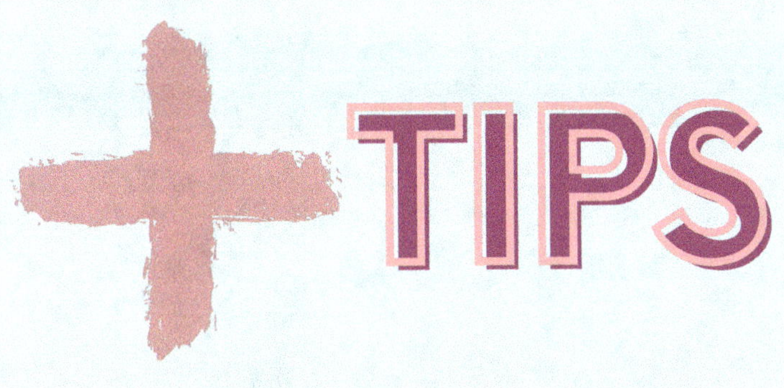

- Find a job or ask your parents how you can earn an allowance
- Schedule 1 or 2 beauty treatments every month. Add on 1 beauty treatment as often as you can
- Read 1 book every month
- Be consistent so that you set a standard for yourself!

Section 3

HYGIENE

HYGIENE

Hygiene is a series of practices performed to preserve health. Hygiene refers to conditions and practices that help to maintain health and prevent the spread of diseases. Personal hygiene refers to maintaining the body's cleanliness. (Wikipedia & World Health Org)

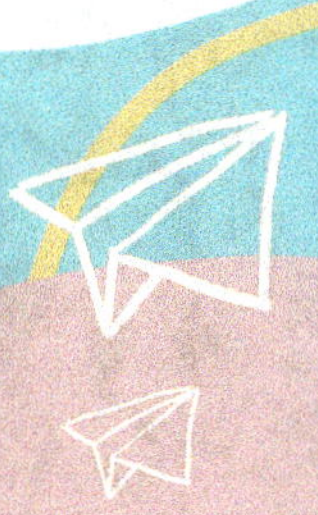

THEMES

1. Preserving Health
2. Preventing Diseases
3. Body Maintenance

WHY DOES GOD EVEN CARE ABOUT THIS STUFF?

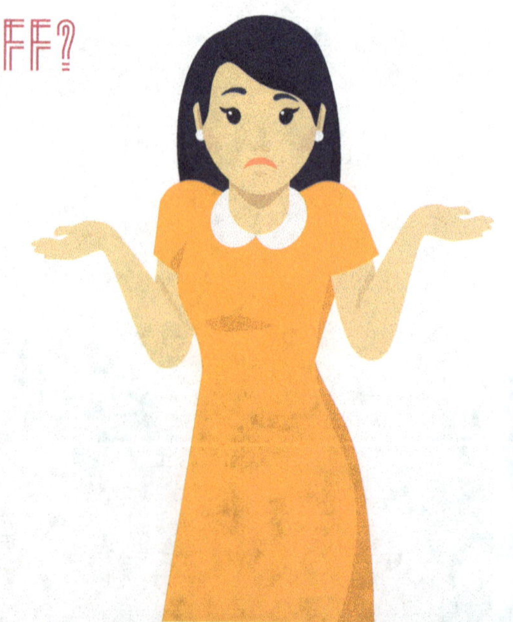

Psalm 139:14
I praise you because I am fearfully and wonderfully made; your works are wonderful, I know that full well.

God cares that we recognize how masterfully he created us! When we look in the mirror and see ourselves as a reflection of God, we praise Him. When we realize that we haven't been taking care of our bodies in ways that reflect our appreciation for how God made us, we take the initiative and watch what we eat or become more disciplined to work out. If we find ourselves always having negative or depressing thoughts, God cares that we take the steps to meditate on the good things in His word. God doesn't want us to get a disease or to spread disease, so He cares how we protect ourselves from dangerous activities and exposures. God cares how we see ourselves because He cares that we see ourselves through how He created us.

preserving health

mental health. physical health. spiritual health.

Here are some things that God says about your mental health...

1 Corinthians 2:16
For who has known the Lord's mind, that he may instruct him? But we have the mind of Christ.

Philippians 2:5-11
5-8 Think of yourselves the way Christ Jesus thought of himself. He had equal status with God but didn't think so much of himself that he had to cling to the advantages of that status no matter what. Not at all. When the time came, he set aside the privileges of deity and took on the status of a slave, became human! Having become human, he stayed human. It was an incredibly humbling process. He didn't claim special privileges. Instead, he lived a selfless, obedient life and then died a selfless, obedient death—and the worst kind of death at that—a crucifixion.

9-11 Because of that obedience, God lifted him high and honored him far beyond anyone or anything, ever, so that all created beings in heaven and on earth—even those long ago dead and buried—will bow in worship before this Jesus Christ, and call out in praise that he is the Master of all, to the glorious honor of God the Father.

Mental Health is a hot topic issue today, it is also a very real public health crisis in our world. Sometimes it seems like "having the mind of Christ" is too simple of a thing to be the solution to all the mental health issues in the world. BUT IT IS! The solution to bad mental health is Christ. We are living in a world that fell to original sin, so everything in it is dying. Christ came so that we all could put our trust in Him that He really did conquer the sin and now has given us a new life to live. Our new life in Christ brings us a new mind to think above all of the issues, problems, and deaths that the world must go through until Christ returns.

If you have anxiousness, worry, sadness, depression, suicidal thoughts, or hopeless thoughts;
1.   Remind yourself that you have the mind of Christ.
2.   Find a trusted someone to talk to about your issues.
3. Meditate on the scriptures above and all of God's word.

Discussion:

What was the last thing you were really anxious, nervous, or depressed about? How did you handle it? Did your solution work?

What will you do the next time you become anxious, nervous, or depressed about something?

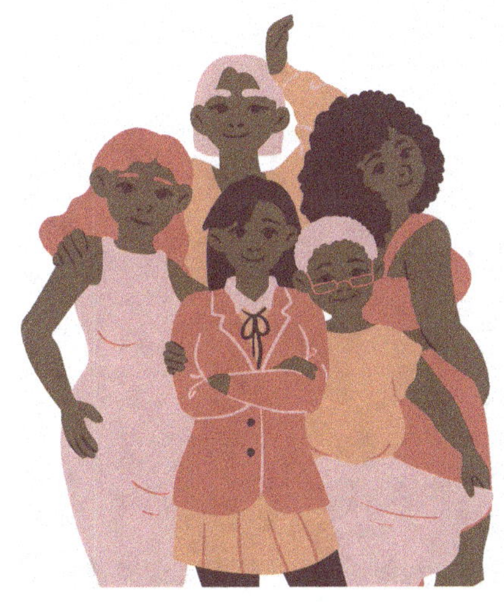

PHYSICAL HEALTH

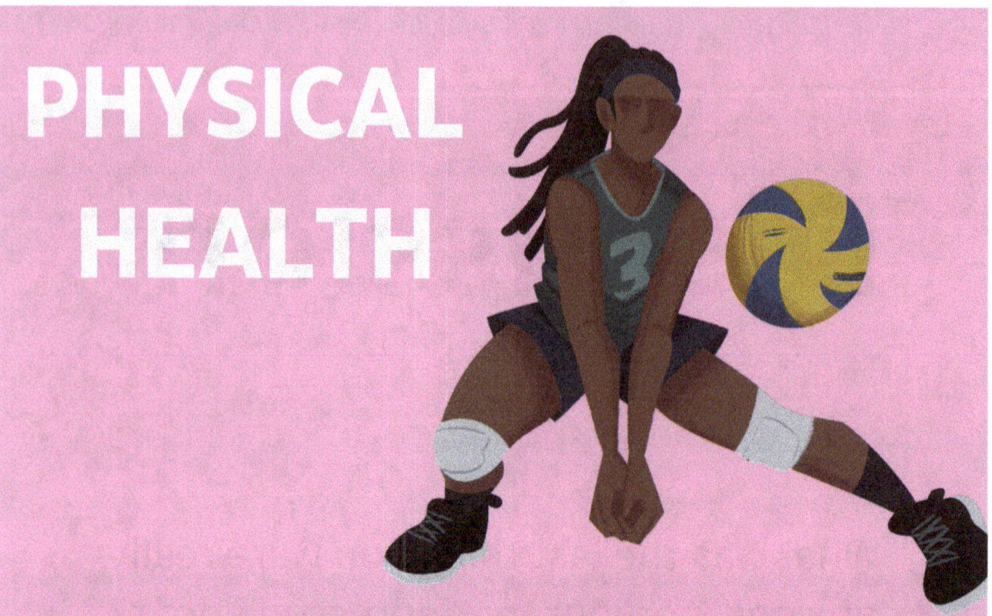

IN TODAY'S WORLD PHYSICAL APPEARANCE TAKES CENTER STAGE ON SOCIAL MEDIA AND AT SCHOOL.

BUT, WE SHOULD NOT OBSESS ABOUT OUR OUTWARD APPEARANCE, WE SHOULD MAKE THE EFFORT TO STAY FIT BECAUSE IT HELPS US TO DEVELOP DISCIPLINE.

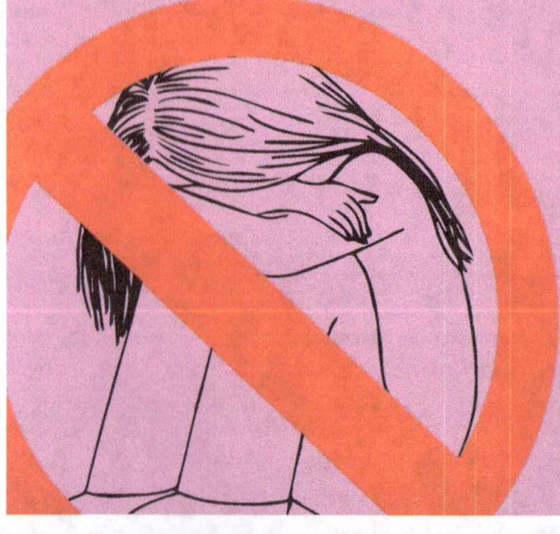

YOUR SHAPE; YOUR BEAUTY; YOUR FLAWS; OR YOUR APPEARANCE IS NEVER AN INVITATION FOR SOMEONE ELSE TO ATTACK OR MISUSE FOR THEIR SATISFACTION.

As females, you must learn to be kind and firm. If God didn't say it about you, its ok for you to reject it as opinion, a possible fact, or a total lie. Do not continue to meditate on others comments about you that make you feel insecure or less than. Smile, say thank you for your comment, and move on to better people.

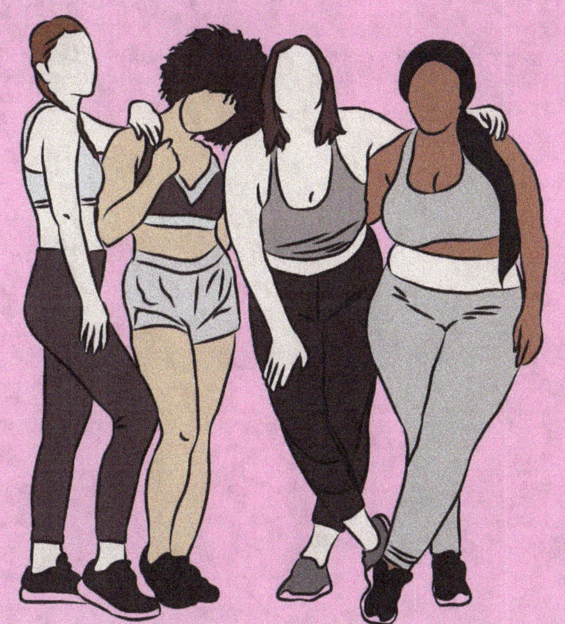

Preventing Disease

Ways Infectious diseases spread

- air as small droplets
- contact with feces (poo) and then with the mouth
- contact with the skin or mucus membranes (nose, mouth, throat, and genitals)
- blood or other body fluids (sexual contact)

(Ministry of Health NZ)

We all have a responsibilty to guard our bodies against diseases. Prayer is our first line of defense but we need to back it up with actions of faith including;

- wearing face masks
- vaccines (if led by the Lord)
- using hand sanitizer and washing our hands frequently
- remaining safe distances from people; avoiding unnecessary contact
- abstinence

Body Maintenance

FOCUS: ABSTINENCE

noun: the fact or practice of restraining oneself from indulging in something; typically alcohol.

> But if you do not do what is right, sin is crouching at your door; it desires to have you, but you must rule over it."
>
> GENESIS 4:6-7

A simple word for abstinence is self-control. Remember, you are God's daughter who He has made uniquely special. He created you to solve problems. One thing that you will always face is temptation to bring more problems in your life- which will distract you from solving problems.

By employing self-control and abstinence you will dominate every temptation of alcoholism, drug-abuse, mental health issues, and premature sexual relationships that can ruin your life if you try to indulge at an early age.

DISCUSSION:
God created you to solve problems in your generation. What are some things that can prevent you or delay you from walking in your purpose?

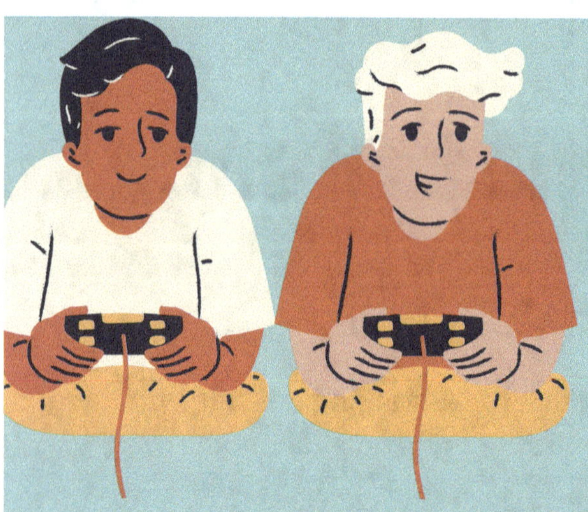

BOYS, BOYS, BOYS

They are cute, annoying, active, and powerful. Let's discuss how to understand boys and how girl and boy power should work together!

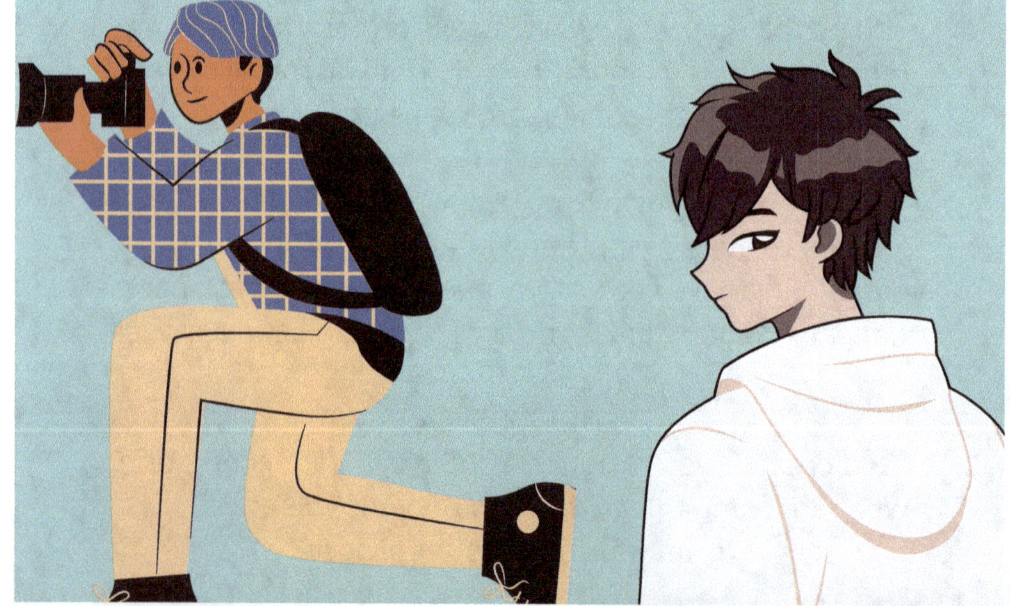

The boys in the bible were not perfect AT ALL. Us girls
can find perfect peace in knowing that the only
perfect male to walk the earth was Jesus.

LET'S TAKE A LOOK AT A FEW OF THE BOYS IN THE BIBLE AND HOW GOD USED THEM....

ADAM

Flaws: He was disobedient by listening to his wife and not God.
Usefulness: Hard worker and a great father to teach his children
to honor God.

ABRAHAM

Flaws: a liar, scaredy-cat, and idol- worshipper
Usefulness: A great Father of faith; He believed everything God
told him and obeyed.

JACOB

Flaws: a deceiver
Usefulness: He was the father of the 12 tribes of Israel.

KING DAVID

Flaws: was a murderer.
Usefulness: He had a heart after God.

APOSTLE PETER

Flaws: hot-tempered, arrogant, and a denier of Jesus
Usefulness: Jesus restored him and sent him out to be an apostle
to care for and feed the church

APOSTLE PAUL

Flaws: a persecuter of Jesus
Usefulness: Jesus converted him and used him to write most of
the New Testament.

boys are created to model leadership...

Leaders can also be girls but God chose to demonstrate what leadership should look like through the male character. Males were created to lead families. Leaders are called to take the responsibility and blame over those they lead. Leaders are also given the rewards of great leadership. Learn to see and treat males as leaders. A few simple ways to honor them could be:

- listen to them
- hold them accountable to do what they promise or if they cause any harm
- encourage them if they struggle in certain areas
- encourage them to seek God for direction
- celebrate them

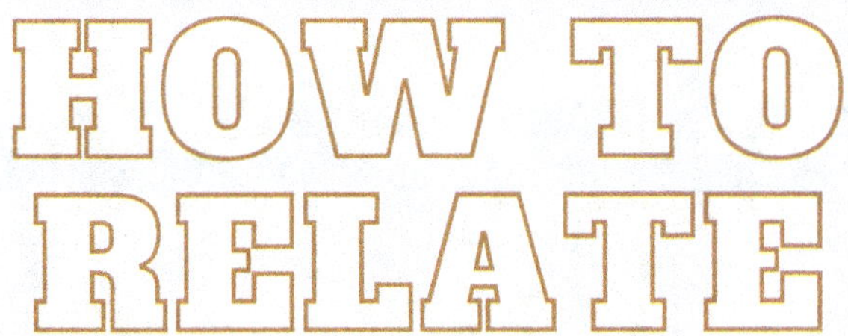

During tween/teen years it can be difficult to sort through relationships with our girlfriends let alone boys. But believe it or not, it is very possible to have thriving, appropriate, and meaningful relationships with boys. It all starts with honoring God, being secure in who He created you to be, and honoring the males in your life.

If you learn to dishonor males in your life, you will not have good relationships with males who are your peers.

HOW DOES HONOR WORK?

Honor is demonstrated by placing others above ourselves.

Romans 12:10: Love one another with brotherly affection. Outdo one another in showing honor.

Females were created to be helpers. We have a beautiful ability and gifting to empower, encourage, nurture, and help others to be successful. God purposefully created you female to ensure that others would benefit from your unique ability to honor and serve others in ways that only you can do!

HONOR ISN'T

- Allowing boys in your life to abuse your friendship.
- Allowing boys in your life to convince you to have sex with them.
- Encouraging boys in your life to hurt themselves by using drugs or alcohol
- Helping boys in your life go down destructive paths; encouraging violence or other activities that go against God
- Manipulating, using, and bossing boys around to get the things that you want out of them.

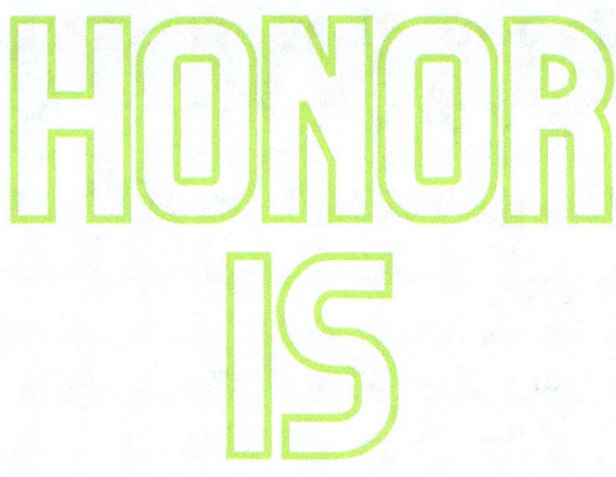

- **learning to appreciate and value your male friendships**
- **to find qualities in your male friends that you respect and admire**
- **to build the kind of trust with males that will allow you to obey and follow them in good ways**
- **allow boys to encourage you and be a safe friend in your life.**

TIP: don't be afraid of the word SUBMIT when it comes to males. Learning healthy submission will benefit you in school, work, and marriage. Submission is an act of faith to submit under the order and authority of another.

What about boys that are struggling with sexual identity or whether or not they are gay? How can I be a friend?

This is a very important question and situation in our culture today. You may find yourself friends with a male who doesn't know if he is a "he" or wants to explore his sexuality. Again, you must be secure in who God made you to be so your first step is to ask the Lord if He desires for you to remain close friends with this person. Why?

Jesus is Lord in the life of a believer, therefore He knows where He is leading you. He may not be leading you to friendship with someone struggling with sin in this way. If He is not leading you, you will find yourself ill-equipped to truly be a friend to the person and likely struggling with compromise or even being overtaken by the person's sin. The best way to be a friend may be to not be a close friend or a friend at all.

If you are a strong believer (read/study/pray God's word) and not easily influenced by the world, you may be the perfect friend for this person- Jesus will let you know. He will give you words to encourage and pray for this person while being a trusted friend in their life. You will know in your heart that the friendship has nothing to do with you, and may not benefit you at all, but that God is using you to keep that person close to Him.

Again, in both cases- Jesus is making the decision and provisions for the friendship. Prayer is the first step to all successful relationships.

Proverbs 27:9
Sweet friendships refresh the soul and awaken our hearts with joy, for good friends are like the anointing oil that yields the fragrant incense of God's presence.

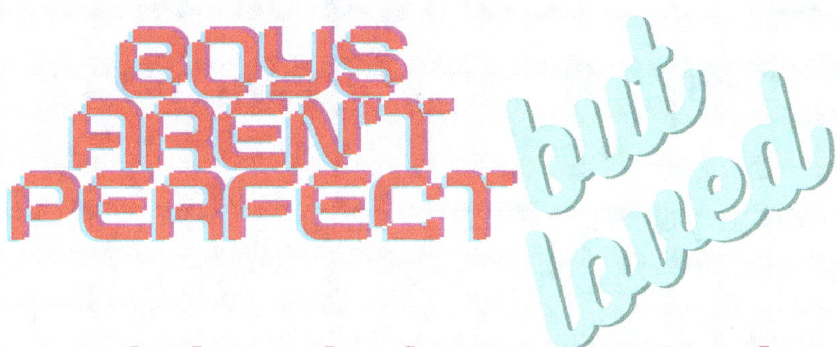

and they belong to God and he can use them!

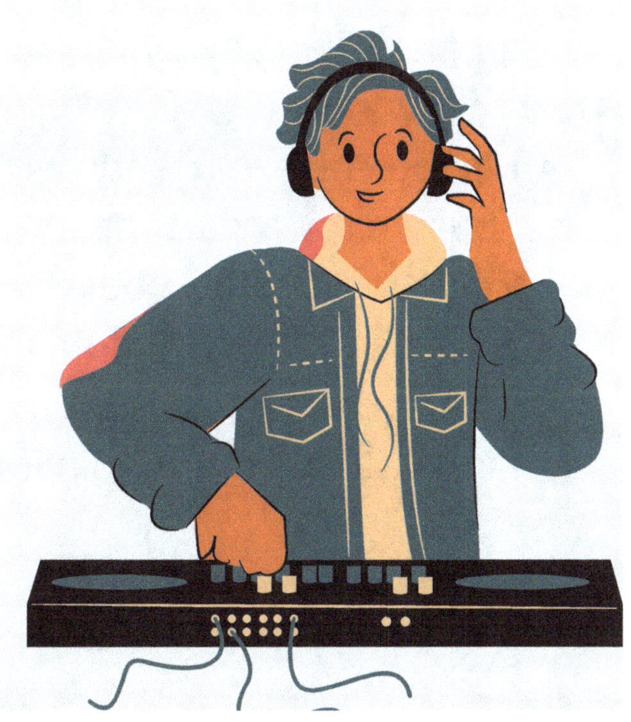

Questions to pray about when it comes to friendship with boys.

- Maybe you are attracted to a boy and thinking of having sex? Ask the Lord to help you walk in the authority you have over temptation.

- Maybe you want to be friends with a male, but he is always caught up in trouble. Ask the Lord the best way to be a positive influence in his life. (*sometimes this may mean walking away)

- Maybe you are friends with a boy who is abusive toward others and or himself. Begin praying for your friend and that God would set him free from abuse. Seek a parent or trusted adult to help you navigate this friendship in a godly manner.

SECTION 5
WINNING THE BATTLE

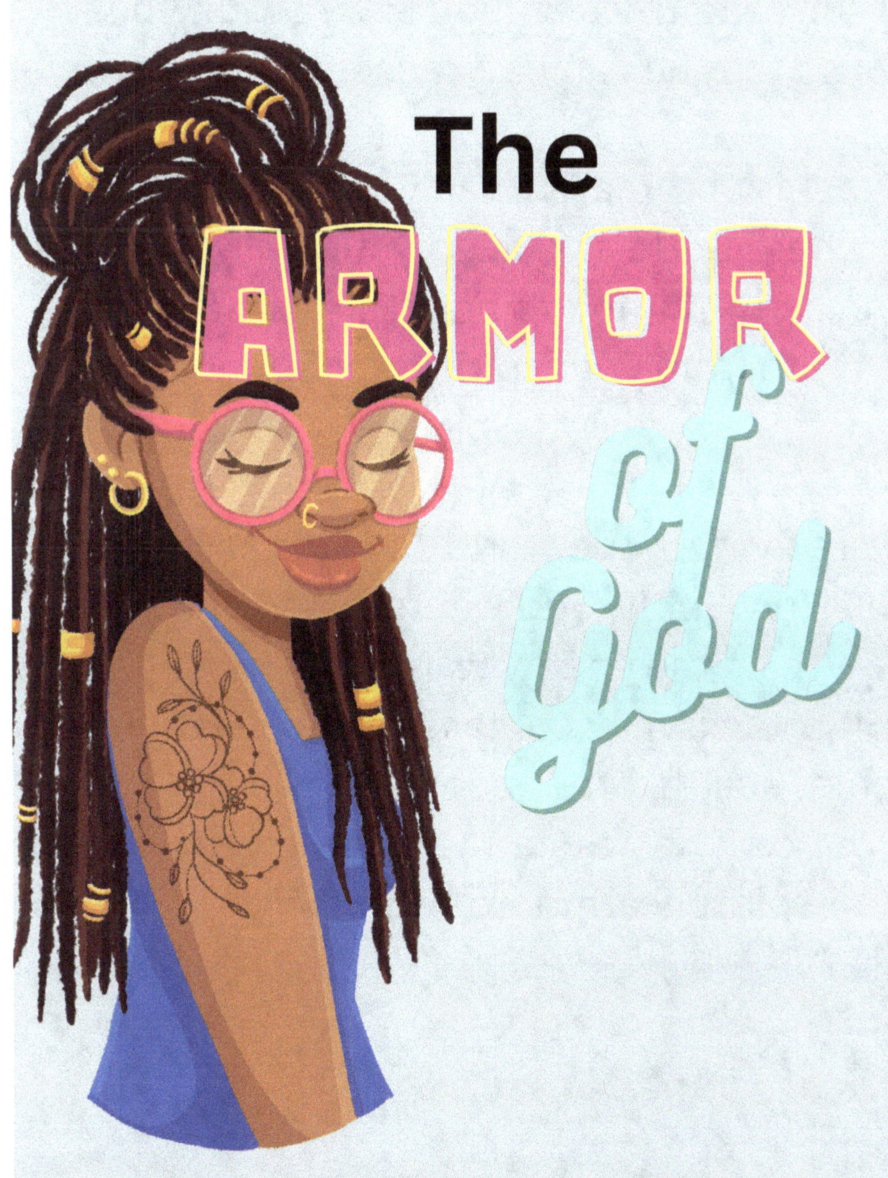

Did you know that you are in a war? The war is for the possession of your soul. Your soul includes your mind, will, and emotions. The enemy, satan, wants you to live from your soul so that he can have access to your life.

Your spirit is greater than your soul and it is where God has placed your ability to correctly live and to hear Him. He directs your life from your spirit by giving you The Holy Spirit.

We are living in the world so with the help of the Holy Spirit, God wants us to conquer everything the enemy wants to throw at us. His attacks may come through negative mental health, other people, or from within our own hearts- but God has given us spiritual armor to help us fight!

The belt of truth.

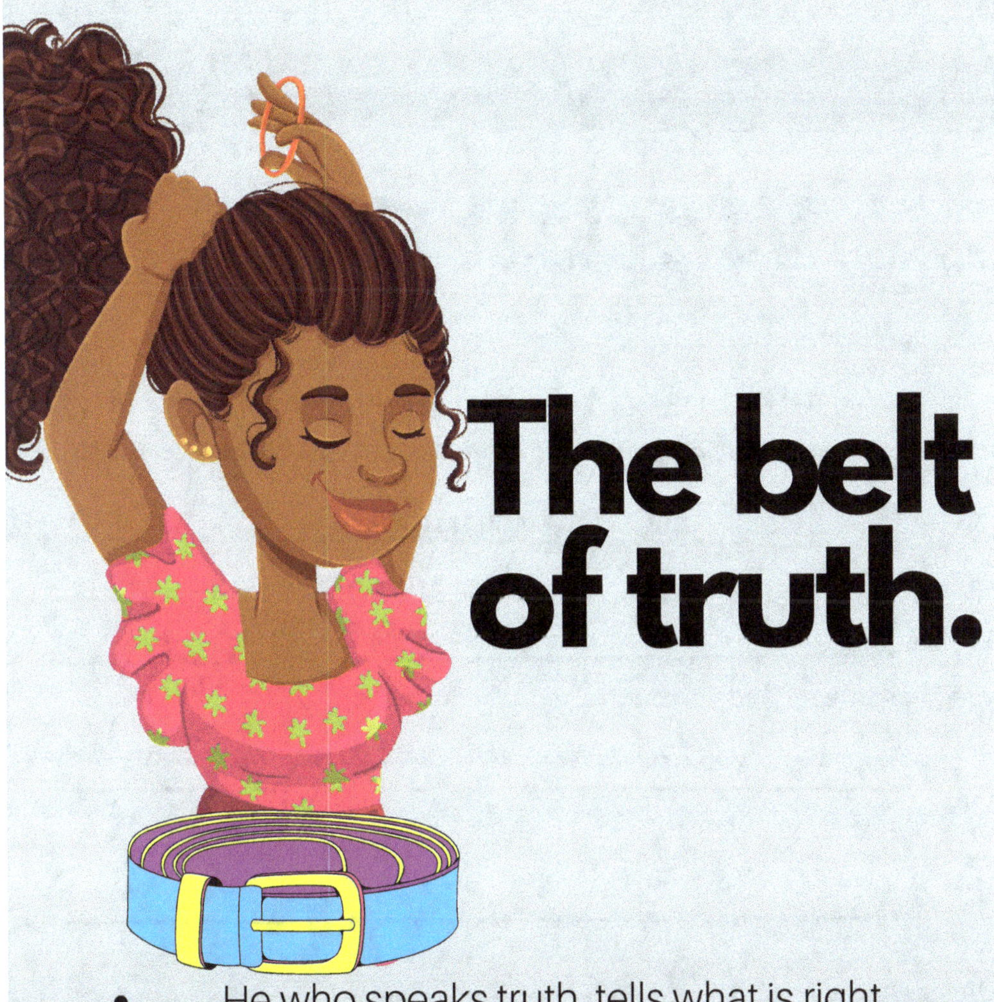

- He who speaks truth, tells what is right. (Proverbs 12:17)
- Jesus said, I am the way the truth and the life; no one comes to the Father but through Me. (John 14:6)
- And youy will know the truth, and the truth will make you free. (John 8:32)

Work It Out:

1. A belt is used to hold up your pants. How does "truth" hold you up when all is going wrong?

____

____

____

____

____

____

- But seek first the kingdom of God and His righteousness, and all these things shall be added to you. (Matthew 6:33)
- Many are the afflictions of the righteous, but the Lord delivers him out of them all. (Psalm 34:19)
- A man is not established by wickedness, but the root of the righteous cannot be moved. (Proverbs 12:3)

the breastplate of righteousness

Work It Out:

1. **What are the benefits to you and others if you guard your heart with a righteous breastplate?**

____

____

____

____

____

____

HELMET

of Salvation

- **Salvation comes no other way; no other name has been or will be given to us by which we can be saved, only this one. (Acts 4:12)**

- **Let this mind be in you, which was also in Christ Jesus. (Philippians 2:5)**

- **We tear down barriers erected against the truth of God, and we are taking every thought and purpose captive to the obedience of Christ. (2 Corinthians 10:5)**

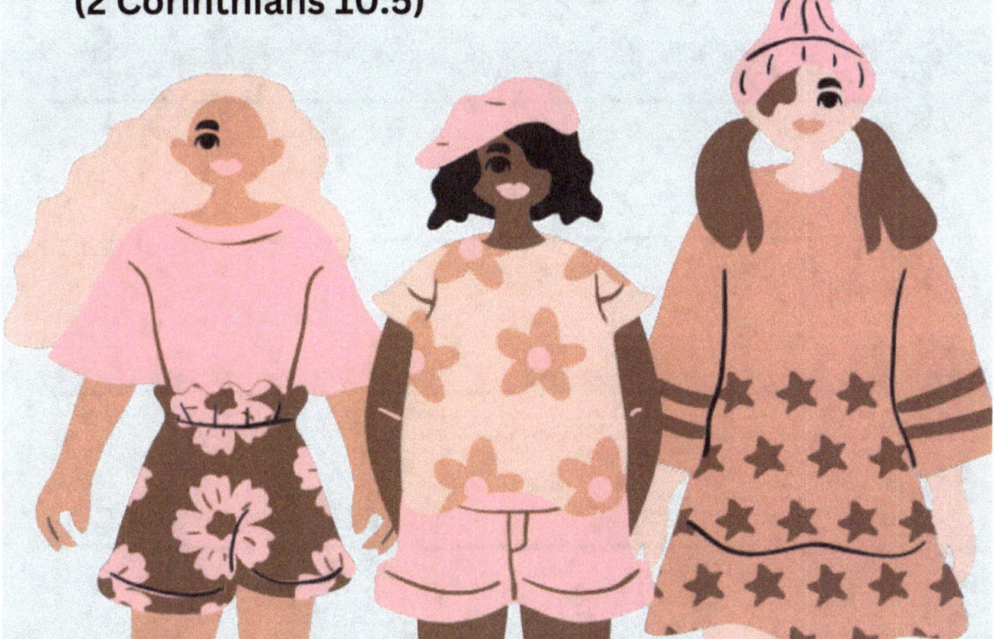

Work It Out:

1. **What are some ideas and ways in the world that you wonder is against God?**

____

____

____

____

____

____

____

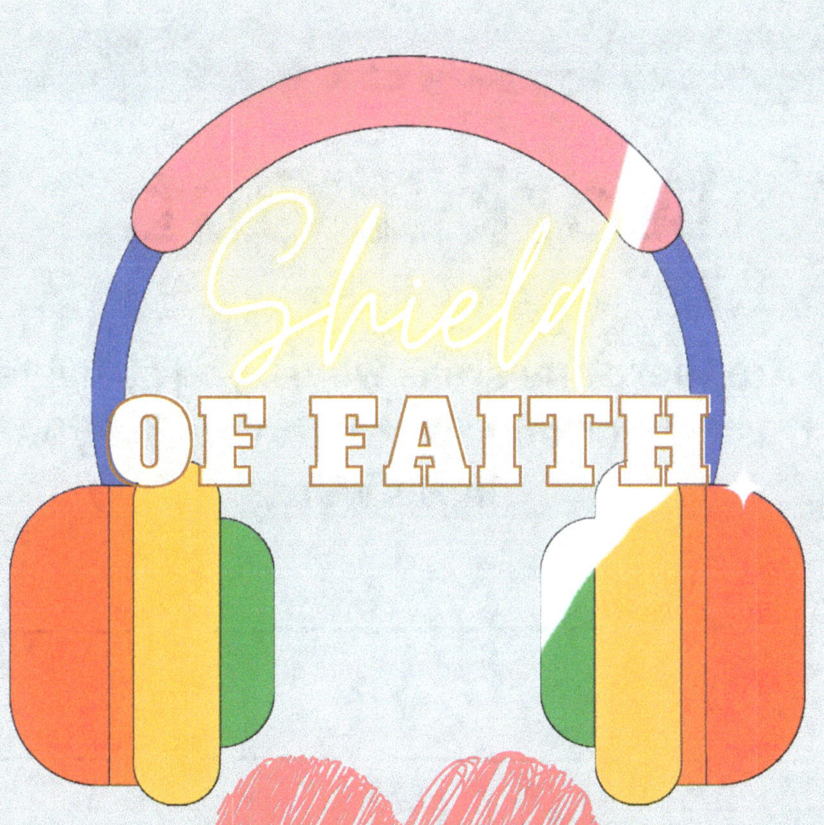

- **So faith comes from hearing and hearing through the word of Christ. (Romans 10:17)**
- **For we walk by faith, not by sight.**
- **(2 Corinthians 5:7)**
- **So that your faith might not rest in the wisdom of men but in the power of God. (1 Corinthians 2:5)**

Work It Out:

1. Are there any areas where you struggle to trust what God says about you and your life in His word?

____

____

____

____

____

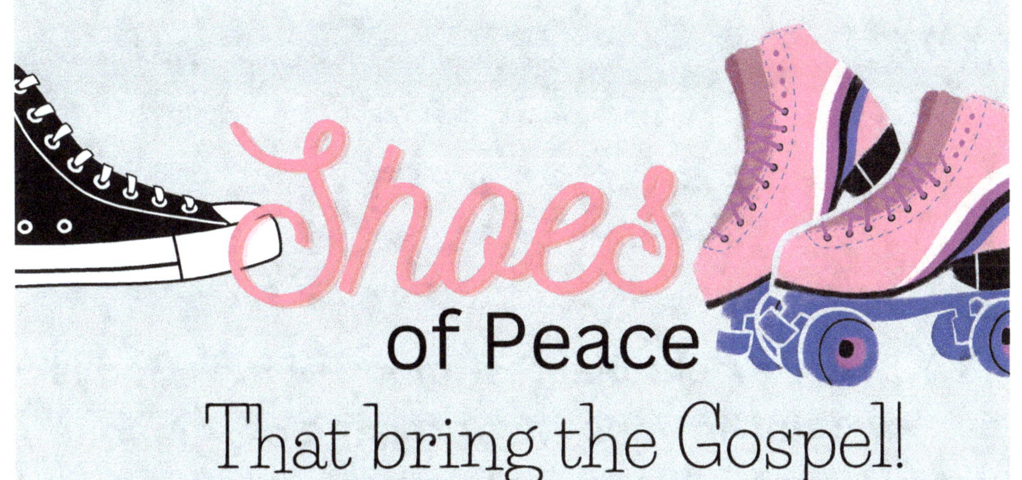

Shoes of Peace
That bring the Gospel!

- For God so loved the world that he gave his only begotten son, that whosoever believes in him shall not perish but have everlasting life. (John 3:17)

- This is eternal life: that they may know You, the only true God, and the One you have sent- Jesus Christ. (John 17:3)

- The thief comes but only to steal, kill and to destroy! I am come that they might have life, and that they might have it more abundantly. (John 10:10)

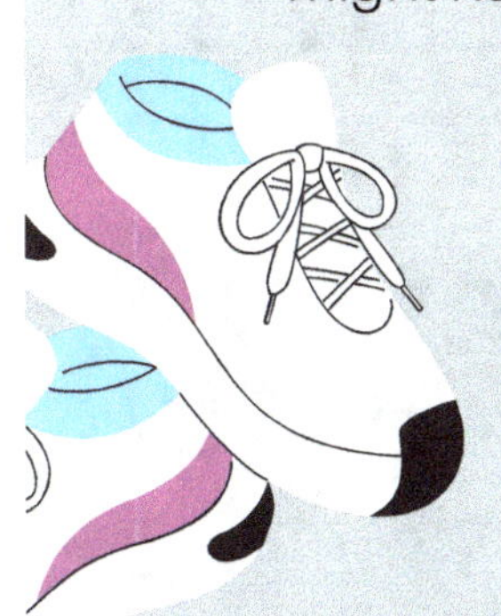

Work It Out:

1. **Share a personal testimony of how God is working in your life or the life of someone you know.**

____

____

____

____

____

Sword of the Spirit

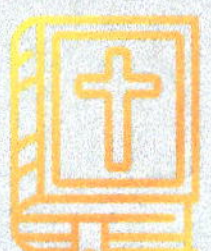

Matthew 4:4-11...

But Jesus said, "It is written, Man is not to live on bread only. Man is to live by every word that God speaks."

Jesus said to the devil, "It is written also, You must not tempt the Lord your God.

Jesus said, Get away Satan. It is written, You must worship the Lord your God. you must obey Him only.

Then the devil went away from Jesus. Angels came and cared for Him.

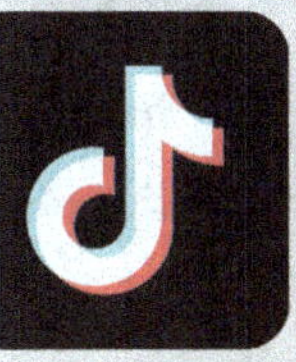
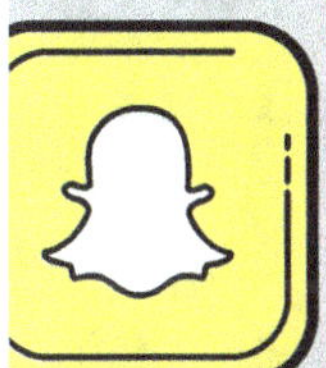

Work It Out:

If a friend on social media was battling depression or suicidal thoughts, what scripture do you think you would share as a social media post?

____

____

____

____

FAMILY

GENESIS 18:19
FOR I HAVE CHOSEN HIM, THAT HE MAY COMMAND HIS
CHILDREN AND HIS HOUSEHOLD AFTER HIM TO KEEP THE WAY
OF THE LORD BY DOING RIGHTEOUSNESS AND JUSTICE, SO THAT
THE LORD MAY BRING TO ABRAHAM WHAT HE HAS PROMISED
HIM.

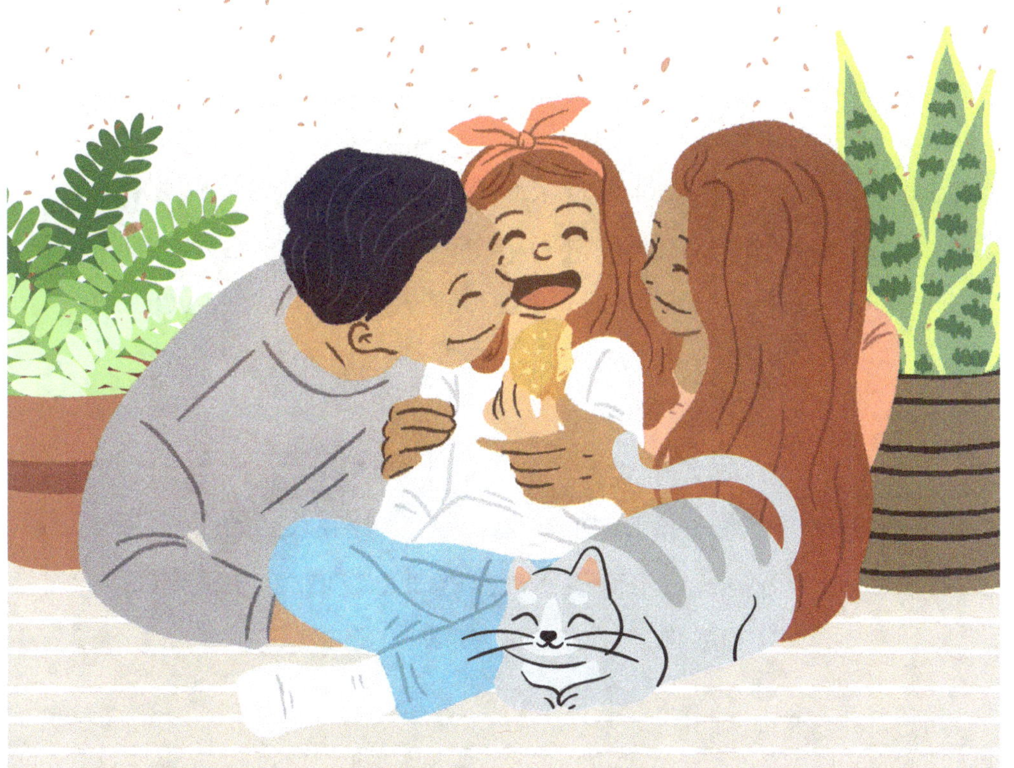

One of the first wonderful things that we learn about God is that He loves creating families! In creation, He formed families of animals and birds; plants and trees; and finally humans. His purpose for human families is to help one another and produce children that fear God and live righteously

You were born into a family with a purpose and on purpose. God knew exactly who your parents were going to be; any issues or troubles you would face in the family; all of the celebrations and accomplishments that would happen in your family; and the uniqueness you would bring to your family dynamic.

You aren't living by coincidence or accident. You were a planned member of your family and God has His eye on you and wants you to discover and live out the plan he made for you to impact your family in ways that only you can do!

In this chapter, we are going to break down the roles within the family, how to embrace your role, and how God sees the different kinds of families within our societies today.

Family Roles

Fathers are to know the ways and commands of God. They are to follow Him while leading his family; protecting his family; providing for his family; and overseeing the welfare of his family. God gives fathers the vision for the family. Father's must also be good joke tellers!

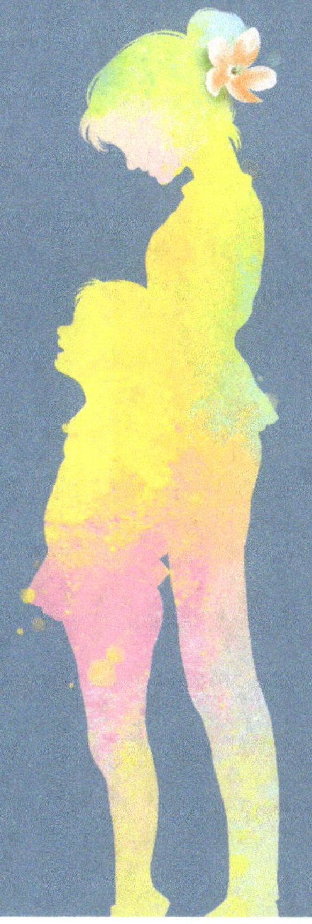

Mothers are the teachers who helps the family by executing and managing the vision for the family. Mother's largely influence and help to shape the character of her children. Moms are expected to pray for their families and serve them as unto the Lord. Mother's are the great warriors for family success!

Honor your father and your mother, that your days may be long in the land that the Lord your God is giving you.

EXODUS 20:12

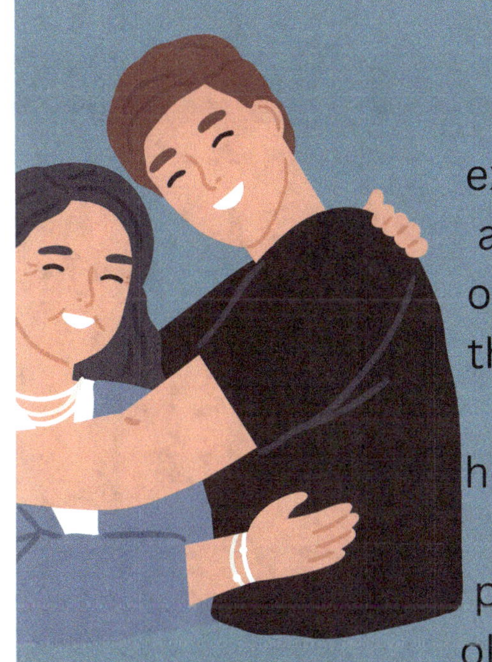

Sons are a beautiful expression of the future of a man's family. He carries on the name and builds on the legacy and adds to the vision. Sons lead in honoring their parents and helps to take care of his parents once they are too old to care for themselves.

Daughters are a blessing to her family and add value wherever she goes. She brings a nurturing spirit, optimism, and grace to every situation. She carries with her the best qualities of a family and is favored wherever she goes.

embracing
your role

God sets the lonely in
families.

Behold, children are a
heritage from the Lord, the
fruit of the womb a reward.
Like arrows in the hand of a
warrior are the children of
one's youth. Blessed is the
man who fills his quiver with
them! He shall not be put to
shame when he speaks with
his enemies in the gate.

Answer these questions...

1. What unique qualities do you bring to your family?

2. What qualities do you like best about your parents?

3. What are some ways that you can continue to deposit your significance in your family?

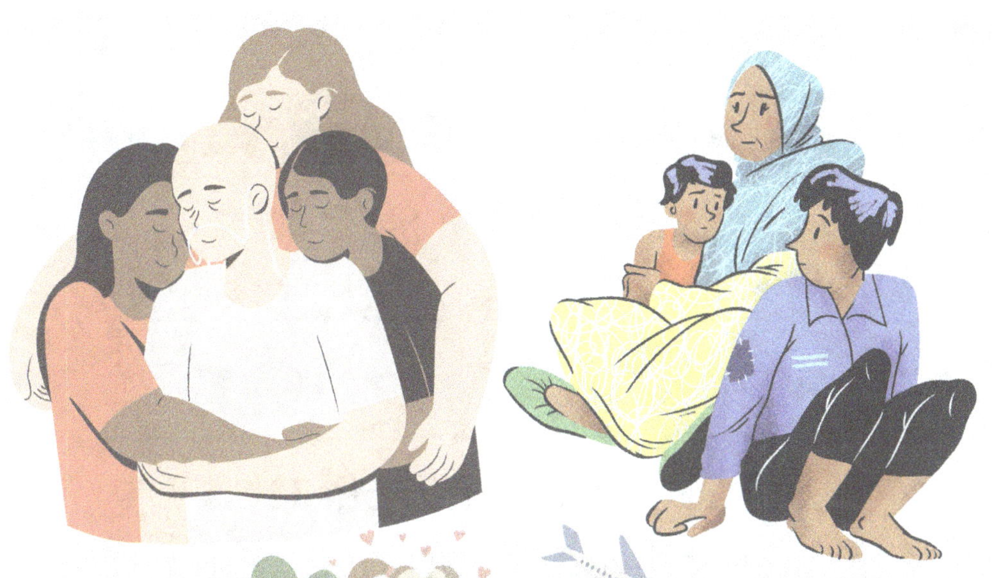

Different kinds of families in our world

TRADITIONAL FAMILIES
BLENDED FAMILIES
SAME-SEX FAMILIES
SINGLE PARENT FAMILIES

30 Love the Lord your God with all your heart and with all your soul and with all your mind and with all your strength.'[a] 31 The second is this: 'Love your neighbor as yourself.'[b] There is no commandment greater than these."

MARK 12:30-31

Let's Talk About it!!!!

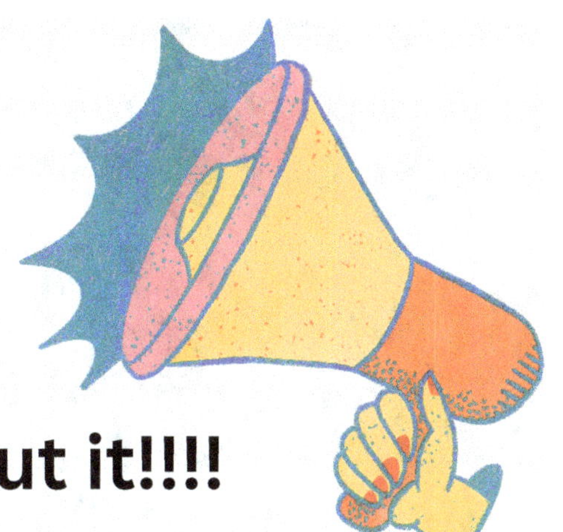

If you live on earth, there is no way to miss that there are many types of families in our neighborhoods. Christians honor God's order for family and believe in man and woman led families/households. Believers in Christ are called to follow the ways of the Lord and be separate from what others may be doing as far as family is concerned; but this doesn't mean that you can't love and respect others because of their family structure.

Jesus was so wise because he knew that we would struggle with living with one another so he gives us two commandments to follow, "love the Lord God with all our heart, mind and strength and love our neighbors as we love ourselves." Loving ourselves includes us wanting the best for ourselves; wanting to live in peace; and wanting to be a blessing. This is the same love we must be willing to forward to our neighbors no matter how their family is structured.

If you find it difficult to love your neighbor because maybe they have a household with 2 dads instead of a mom and a dad; the best way to love them is to leave them alone until God can work genuine love into your heart for them that pours His love from you to them.

These scriptures will help you understand how God wants us to live among different family types.

1 Thessalonians 5:15–18, NLT See that no one pays back evil for evil, but always try to do good to each other and to all people. Always be joyful. Never stop praying. Be thankful in all circumstances, for this is God's will for you who belong to Christ Jesus.

Romans 15:5, MSG May our dependably steady and warmly personal God develop maturity in you so that you get along with each other as well as Jesus gets along with us all.

Hebrews 12:14, NIV Make every effort to live in peace with everyone and to be holy; without holiness no one will see the Lord.

know what
you believe...

and why you
believe it

JUDE 3 PROJECT

Journaling Activity:

Are there any family structure that you have questions about? List them and discuss with your group.

____

____

____

____

____

____

YOU DID IT!

Thank you for being a crucial part of It's A Girl Thing Movement! Our hope is to get you excited and comfortable about what makes you a unique daughter of God in Christ! We hope that your gifts have been stirred and your love for God has been increased!

Continue to seek Him with all of your questions, concerns, doubts, and needs...don't let fear hold you back from getting all of the treasures and wealth of knowledge and understanding that Jesus gave his life for you to find. He did an AMAZING work for your benefit!

Stay connected with the movement through our YouTube page @ministryalliancelove We post shorts for you to share and offer workshops to help you on your journey in Christ.

Blessings to you always!